Copyright 2023 Olivia G Louis

Table of contents

Chapter 1. Understanding Binge Eating

- What is Binge Eating?
- The Cycle of Binge Eating

Chapter 2. Recognizing Triggers

- Emotional Triggers
- Environmental Triggers
- Social Triggers

Chapter 3. Mindful Eating Practices

- Intuitive Eating
- Mindful Eating Techniques
- Developing a Healthy Relationship with Food

Chapter 4. Building a Support System

- Seeking Professional Help
- Finding Support Groups
- Enlisting Friends and Family Support

Chapter 5. Coping Strategies

- Stress Management Techniques
- Healthy Distractions
- Relaxation and Meditation

Chapter 6. Developing Healthy Habits

- Meal Planning and Preparation
- Balanced Nutrition
- Regular Exercise

Chapter 7. Overcoming Emotional Eating

- Understanding Emotions and Food
- Finding Alternative Coping Mechanisms
- Cognitive Behavioral Techniques

Chapter 8. Maintaining Progress and Preventing Relapse

- Staying Committed to Recovery
- Identifying Warning Signs
- Strategies for Long-Term Success

Chapter 1

Understanding Binge Eating

- ## What is Binge Eating?

A persistent episode of consuming a lot of food in a short amount of time, along with a feeling of losing control over eating behaviour, is what defines binge eating disorder (BED), a serious eating disorder. BED binge eating episodes are not followed by compensatory behaviours like purging, excessive exercise, or fasting, in contrast to other eating disorders like anorexia nervosa or bulimia nervosa.

1. Characteristics of Binge Eating:

- **Consuming Large Amounts of Food:** During binge eating episodes, individuals typically eat much larger amounts of food than most people would under similar circumstances. This can include consuming large quantities of high-calorie, high-fat, or high-sugar foods.
- **Loss of Control:** The inability to quit eating during an episode of binge eating is one of its defining characteristics. People frequently describe feeling as though they are eating on autopilot and are not in control

of what they are doing.
• Rapid Eating: During periods of binge eating, eating frequently takes place quickly, with little time spent truly appreciating the flavour and texture of the food.
• Emotional Distress: During and after a binge eating episode, feelings of guilt, shame, or distress are frequently experienced. This psychological discomfort has the potential to worsen the binge eating pattern and fuel depressive and low-self-esteem sentiments.

2. Frequency and Duration:

- To satisfy the diagnostic requirements for BED, binge eating episodes must occur at least once a week on average for three months. However, there can be significant individual variation in the frequency and intensity of binge eating episodes..
- Binge eating episodes may last for a few minutes to several hours, depending on individual circumstances and triggers.

3. Triggers for Binge Eating:

- **Emotional Triggers:** Emotional Triggers: A lot of people with BED say they turn to food to help them deal with challenging feelings like stress, melancholy, boredom, or loneliness. Emotional distress can be momentarily distracted from or soothed by

binge eating.
• Environmental Triggers: Being around particular foods, feeling overstimulated by food-related activities or social gatherings, or feeling especially stressed out at work or school are some examples of environmental signals or conditions that can set off binge eating episodes.

- **Dieting and Restriction:** Restrictive dieting and attempts to control food intake can paradoxically increase the likelihood of binge eating episodes. This is often referred to as the "diet-binge cycle," where periods of strict dieting are followed by episodes of binge eating due to feelings of deprivation and loss of control.

4. Impact on Physical and Mental Health:

- The effects of binge eating can be detrimental to one's physical and emotional well-being. It can exacerbate physical health concerns such as heart disease, diabetes, obesity, weight gain, and other disorders.
• Binge eating disorders can have a severe emotional toll, resulting in depressive, guilty, ashamed, and self-loathing feelings.

5. Treatment and Recovery:
- Binge eating disorder is a treatable condition, and recovery is possible with the right support and interventions. Treatment

> approaches may include cognitive-behavioral therapy (CBT), interpersonal therapy, dialectical behavior therapy (DBT), nutritional counseling, and medication.
>
> - Support groups, online forums, and peer support networks can also be valuable resources for individuals seeking recovery from binge eating disorder.

Binge eating is a complex and challenging eating disorder characterized by recurrent episodes of consuming large amounts of food accompanied by a sense of loss of control. It can have serious physical and emotional consequences, but with the right support and treatment, individuals can learn to manage their symptoms and achieve long-term recovery.

The cycle of binge eating refers to the repetitive pattern of behaviors, emotions, and thoughts that often characterize binge eating disorder (BED) and contribute to its perpetuation. Understanding this cycle is crucial for individuals struggling with BED and for healthcare professionals providing treatment and support. Usually, the cycle comprises four primary phases:

The Cycle of Binge Eating

1. Triggering Event:

The cycle often begins with a triggering event or situation that prompts the individual to turn to food as a coping mechanism. Triggers can vary widely and may include emotional stress, interpersonal conflict, boredom, loneliness, low self-esteem, or exposure to certain foods or environments associated with previous binge eating episodes.

2. Emotional and Cognitive Responses:

In response to the trigger, the individual experiences a range of emotional and cognitive responses. These may include feelings of anxiety, sadness, anger, frustration, or a sense of emptiness. Negative thoughts and beliefs about oneself, body image, or food may also intensify during this phase. The individual may feel overwhelmed by emotions and may perceive food as a source of comfort, distraction, or control.

3. Binge Eating Episode:

The emotional and cognitive distress experienced during the triggering event leads to a loss of control over eating behavior, triggering a binge eating episode. During the binge, the individual consumes large quantities of food rapidly, often in secret and to the point of discomfort. Despite feelings of guilt, shame, or disgust, the individual feels unable to stop eating or control their behavior. The binge eating episode provides temporary relief from emotional distress but is followed by intense feelings of regret and self-recrimination.

4. Post-Binge Consequences:

The person has a variety of physical and psychological after-binge effects when the binge eating session passes. Overindulging in food can cause physical discomfort such bloating, indigestion, and fatigue. Emotionally, the person might feel more guilty, ashamed, or self-loathing, which would exacerbate any unfavourable self-perceptions they already had and their capacity to regulate their eating habits. These unfavourable feelings frequently prolong the binge eating pattern because people may revert to eating in order to manage the emotional pain brought on by the binge and the ensuing low opinion of themselves.

Breaking the Cycle:

Breaking the cycle of binge eating requires targeted interventions aimed at addressing the underlying triggers, emotions, and behaviors associated with the disorder. Cognitive-behavioral therapy (CBT), dialectical behavior therapy (DBT), interpersonal therapy, and mindfulness-based approaches are commonly used in the treatment of binge eating disorder. These therapies help individuals develop healthier coping mechanisms for managing emotions, challenging negative thought patterns, improving self-esteem, and fostering a more balanced relationship with food.

Apart from counselling, alterations in lifestyle including meal planning on a regular basis, maintaining a healthy diet, getting enough sleep, managing stress, and indulging in enjoyable hobbies can also aid in the recovery process from binge eating disorder. Building a strong support network of friends, family, and healthcare professionals can provide encouragement, accountability, and practical assistance throughout the recovery process.

Overall, breaking the cycle of binge eating requires a comprehensive and individualized approach that addresses the complex interplay of psychological, emotional, and behavioral factors contributing to the disorder. People can learn to control their symptoms, create healthy coping mechanisms, and achieve long-term recovery from binge eating disorder with commitment, support, and expert advice.

Chapter 2

Recognizing Triggers

- **Emotional Triggers**

The onset and maintenance of eating disorders, including binge eating disorder (BED), are significantly influenced by emotional triggers. These triggers include a broad spectrum of emotional events that might cause people to turn to unhealthy eating habits as a coping mechanism or diversion from painful feelings. Understanding emotional triggers is essential for individuals struggling with BED, as well as for healthcare professionals providing treatment and support.

1. Types of Emotional Triggers:

- **Stress:** Stressful situations at work, school, or home can trigger episodes of binge eating. Individuals may turn to food as a way to cope with feelings of overwhelm, pressure, or anxiety.
- **Sadness and Depression:** Feelings of sadness, hopelessness, or depression can also serve as triggers for binge eating. Food may be used as a temporary source of comfort or distraction from emotional pain.
- **Anger and Frustration:** Intense feelings of anger, frustration, or irritability can lead individuals to seek solace in food. Binge

eating may be used as a means of numbing or suppressing these difficult emotions.

- **Loneliness and Isolation:** Social isolation, feelings of loneliness, or a lack of meaningful connections with others can contribute to binge eating behavior. Food may serve as a companion or surrogate for interpersonal relationships.
- **Boredom:** Monotony or lack of stimulation in daily life can trigger episodes of binge eating. Individuals may turn to food out of boredom or to fill a perceived void in their lives.
- **Low Self-Esteem and Body Image Issues:** Negative beliefs about oneself, body image dissatisfaction, or low self-esteem can fuel feelings of worthlessness or inadequacy, leading individuals to engage in binge eating as a form of self-soothing or validation.

2. Triggers and the Binge Eating Cycle:

Emotional triggers are often intertwined with the binge eating cycle, contributing to a repetitive pattern of maladaptive eating behaviors. People who are exposed to emotional triggers may suffer from increased emotional distress as well as cognitive distortions such illogical ideas about food and body image or negative self-talk. Binge eating episodes can be brought on by these upsetting feelings and ideas, which can lead to a lack of control over eating habits.

During the binge eating episode, individuals may experience temporary relief from emotional discomfort as they engage in compulsive eating behaviors. However, this relief is short-lived and is often followed by intense feelings of guilt, shame, and regret. The negative emotions experienced post-binge can perpetuate the cycle of binge eating, leading individuals to turn to food once again to cope with emotional distress, thus reinforcing the maladaptive pattern of behavior.

3. Strategies for Coping with Emotional Triggers:

Creating healthier coping strategies for handling emotional triggers is necessary to end the binge eating cycle. Among the tactics that could be useful are:

- **Mindfulness and Awareness:** Increasing awareness of emotional triggers and their impact on eating behaviors can empower individuals to make conscious choices and respond to emotions in a more adaptive manner.
- **Emotional Regulation Techniques:** Learning skills for managing emotions, such as deep breathing exercises, progressive

muscle relaxation, and mindfulness meditation, can help individuals cope with emotional distress without resorting to binge eating.

- **Cognitive Restructuring:** Challenging negative thought patterns and replacing them with more realistic and compassionate self-talk can help individuals develop a healthier relationship with themselves and their bodies.
- **Seeking Support:** Building a strong support network of friends, family, support groups, or mental health professionals can provide validation, encouragement, and practical guidance for managing emotional triggers and navigating the recovery process.

By identifying and addressing emotional triggers, individuals can begin to break free from the cycle of binge eating and cultivate more adaptive ways of coping with emotional distress. With time, practice, and support, individuals can develop the resilience and skills necessary to manage their emotions effectively and foster a more balanced and fulfilling relationship with food and themselves.

- **Environmental Triggers**

Environmental triggers refer to external factors and situational cues that can contribute to the onset or exacerbation of binge eating episodes. These triggers encompass various aspects of a person's surroundings, including social, physical, and cultural environments. Understanding environmental triggers is essential for individuals with binge eating disorder (BED) and for healthcare professionals providing support and treatment.

1. Types of Environmental Triggers:

- **Food Availability and Accessibility:** The presence of abundant, high-calorie foods in the environment can serve as a potent trigger for binge eating. Access to vending machines, convenience stores, and fast-food restaurants, as well as the availability of snacks and treats in the home or workplace, can make it easier for individuals to engage in impulsive eating behaviors.
- **Food-Related Events and Social Gatherings:** A lot of food and drink are typically served during social events including parties, celebrations, and family get-togethers. These occasions may cause people to feel compelled to overindulge, tempted, or obligated to eat in front of others, which may cause them to overeat or binge in reaction to social cues.
- **Food Advertising and Media Influence:** The pervasive presence of food advertising, particularly for highly palatable and

indulgent foods, can influence eating behaviors and trigger cravings or urges to binge. Media portrayals of thinness and idealized body images may also contribute to feelings of inadequacy or body dissatisfaction, exacerbating vulnerability to binge eating.

- **Stressful Environments:** High levels of stress at work, school, or home can increase susceptibility to binge eating as a means of coping with emotional distress. Stressful situations, such as deadlines, conflicts, or financial pressures, can trigger cravings for comfort foods or lead to emotional eating as a form of self-soothing or distraction.
- **Cultural and Familial Influences:** Cultural norms, family traditions, and learned eating behaviors can shape individuals' attitudes and behaviors related to food. Family dynamics, mealtime rituals, and cultural celebrations may contribute to patterns of overeating or binge eating within familial or cultural contexts.

2. Impact of Environmental Triggers:

Environmental triggers can exert a powerful influence on eating behaviors, making it difficult for individuals with BED to resist the urge to binge. These triggers can stimulate cravings, override feelings of fullness or satiety, and undermine efforts to maintain balanced and mindful eating habits. Moreover, environmental cues associated with binge eating can reinforce maladaptive patterns of behavior and perpetuate the cycle of binge eating over time.

3. Strategies for Managing Environmental Triggers:

- **Creating a Supportive Environment:** Surrounding oneself with supportive individuals who understand and respect one's struggles with binge eating can provide a sense of validation, encouragement, and accountability. Seeking out social support networks, online communities, or support groups can offer companionship, empathy, and practical guidance for managing environmental triggers.
- **Identifying and Avoiding Triggering Situations:** Recognizing specific environments, situations, or stimuli that trigger binge eating episodes is an important step toward developing strategies for avoidance or mitigation. Avoiding environments where binge foods are readily available, setting boundaries around social gatherings involving food, and practicing assertiveness in saying no to food-related

pressures can help reduce exposure to triggering situations.

- **Developing Coping Skills:** Learning adaptive coping skills for managing stress, emotions, and cravings can empower individuals to respond more effectively to environmental triggers. Techniques such as deep breathing, mindfulness meditation, progressive muscle relaxation, and stress-reduction strategies can help regulate emotions and promote resilience in the face of environmental stressors.

- **Engaging in Alternative Activities:** Distracting oneself with enjoyable or fulfilling activities that provide a sense of pleasure, accomplishment, or relaxation can help shift focus away from food-related triggers. Engaging in hobbies, physical activity, creative pursuits, socializing with friends, or practicing self-care activities can serve as healthy alternatives to binge eating and promote emotional well-being.

By becoming more aware of environmental triggers and developing proactive strategies for managing them, individuals with BED can reduce vulnerability to binge eating and cultivate a healthier relationship with food and their surroundings. With time, practice, and support, individuals can learn to navigate challenging environments more effectively and make progress toward recovery from binge eating disorder.

- **Social Triggers**

Social triggers are external factors originating from interactions with others or societal norms that can influence individuals to engage in binge eating behaviors. These triggers often stem from social situations, relationships, and cultural influences, exerting a significant impact on eating habits and emotional well-being. Understanding social triggers is essential for individuals with binge eating disorder (BED) and for healthcare professionals providing support and treatment.

1. Types of Social Triggers:

- **Social Pressure to Conform:** In social settings such as parties, gatherings, or shared meals, there may be an implicit or explicit pressure to conform to certain eating behaviors or food choices. This pressure can arise from cultural norms, social expectations, or the desire to fit in with peers. Individuals may feel compelled to overeat or binge in order to avoid standing out or to conform to perceived social norms.
- **Food-Centered Events:** Many social occasions revolve around food, such as

holidays, celebrations, or gatherings with friends and family. These events often feature abundant food options, special treats, or traditional dishes that hold cultural or sentimental significance. The presence of tempting foods and the festive atmosphere can trigger cravings and encourage overeating, particularly if food is used as a focal point of social interaction or celebration.

- **Social Comparison:** Observing others' eating behaviors, body sizes, or dietary choices can trigger feelings of comparison, self-consciousness, or inadequacy. Social media platforms, celebrity endorsements, and peer influences can perpetuate unrealistic standards of beauty and promote diet culture messaging, leading individuals to internalize negative beliefs about their own bodies and eating habits. The pressure to measure up to perceived ideals can contribute to feelings of shame, guilt, or dissatisfaction, prompting individuals to seek comfort or validation through binge eating.

- **Emotional Dynamics in Relationships:** Interpersonal relationships, family dynamics, and social interactions can influence individuals' eating behaviors and emotional responses to food. Conflict, stress, or unresolved emotions within relationships may trigger episodes of emotional eating or binge eating as a means of coping with relational challenges or seeking comfort. Conversely, positive social support, validation, and empathy from loved ones can foster resilience and promote healthier coping strategies for managing emotions.

2. Impact of Social Triggers:

Social triggers can elicit a range of emotional responses and cognitive distortions that contribute to the initiation and perpetuation of binge eating episodes. The pressure to conform to social expectations, fear of judgment or rejection, and desire for acceptance or approval from others can undermine individuals' ability to listen to their body's hunger and fullness cues and make autonomous decisions about food intake. Moreover, the shame, guilt, and self-blame that often accompany binge eating episodes can reinforce negative beliefs about oneself and perpetuate the cycle of disordered eating behaviors.

3. Strategies for Managing Social Triggers:

- **Self-Awareness and Mindfulness:** Developing self-awareness of one's triggers, emotions, and reactions to social situations can empower individuals to make conscious choices and respond more effectively to external pressures. Practicing mindfulness techniques, such as deep breathing, grounding exercises, or body scans, can help individuals stay present and attuned to their internal experiences without judgment or reactivity.

- **Setting Boundaries:** Establishing clear boundaries around social situations involving food can help individuals assert their autonomy and prioritize their own well-being. Communicating personal preferences, dietary restrictions, or recovery goals to friends, family members, or hosts can facilitate understanding and respect for individual needs.

- **Cultivating Supportive Relationships:** Surrounding oneself with supportive individuals who validate and affirm one's recovery journey can provide a sense of belonging, encouragement, and accountability. Seeking out support groups, therapy groups, or online communities of individuals with similar experiences can offer companionship, empathy, and practical guidance for navigating social triggers.

- **Developing Coping Skills:** Learning adaptive coping skills for managing stress, emotions, and cravings can empower individuals to respond more effectively to social triggers. Techniques such as cognitive restructuring, problem-solving, and emotion regulation can help individuals challenge negative thought patterns, cope with uncomfortable emotions, and navigate social situations with resilience and self-compassion.

By identifying and addressing social triggers, individuals with BED can develop adaptive coping strategies for managing social pressures, cultivating supportive relationships, and promoting recovery from binge eating disorder. With time, practice, and support, individuals can learn to navigate social situations more effectively and make progress toward building a healthier and more fulfilling relationship with food and themselves.

Chapter 3

Mindful Eating Practices

- **Intuitive Eating**

Intuitive eating is an approach to eating that emphasizes tuning into your body's hunger and fullness cues, honoring your cravings, and cultivating a healthy relationship with food and your body. Developed by dietitians Evelyn Tribole and Elyse Resch, intuitive eating is based on the principle of rejecting diet culture and embracing self-care and body positivity.

1. Principles of Intuitive Eating:

- **Reject the Diet Mentality:** Intuitive eating begins with rejecting the diet mentality, which involves letting go of restrictive eating rules, calorie counting, and the pursuit of weight loss. Instead, intuitive eaters focus on nourishing their bodies and honoring their natural hunger and fullness cues.
- **Honor Your Hunger:** Intuitive eating encourages individuals to listen to their body's hunger signals and respond to them with nourishing foods. By eating when hungry and stopping when full, individuals can maintain a healthy balance of energy

and nutrients without feeling deprived or overly restricted.

- **Make Peace with Food:** All foods are considered morally neutral in intuitive eating, and there are no "good" or "bad" foods. Intuitive eaters are encouraged to give themselves unconditional permission to eat all foods without guilt or judgment. By removing labels of "forbidden" foods, individuals can develop a more relaxed and flexible approach to eating.
- **Challenge the Food Police:** Intuitive eating involves challenging internalized food rules, negative self-talk, and critical thoughts about food and body size. By reframing negative beliefs and practicing self-compassion, individuals can cultivate a more positive and accepting attitude toward themselves and their bodies.
- **Discover the Satisfaction Factor:** Intuitive eating emphasizes the importance of finding pleasure and satisfaction in eating experiences. By savoring flavors, textures, and aromas, individuals can enhance their enjoyment of food and feel more satisfied with smaller portions.
- **Feel Your Fullness:** Intuitive eating encourages individuals to tune into their body's fullness cues and stop eating when satisfied, rather than when overly full or stuffed. By practicing mindful eating and

paying attention to physical sensations of fullness, individuals can develop a greater awareness of their body's signals.

- **Cope with Emotions Without Using Food:** Emotional eating is a common coping mechanism for managing stress, anxiety, sadness, or boredom. Intuitive eating encourages individuals to explore alternative ways of coping with emotions, such as practicing self-care, seeking support from others, or engaging in enjoyable activities.
- **Respect Your Body:** Intuitive eating promotes body acceptance and respect for body diversity. Rather than striving for a specific weight or body shape, individuals focus on nurturing their bodies, appreciating their strengths, and embracing their unique genetic makeup.

2. Benefits of Intuitive Eating:

- **Improved Relationship with Food:** Intuitive eating helps individuals develop a more positive and balanced relationship with food, free from guilt, shame, and anxiety.
- **Enhanced Body Awareness:** By tuning into hunger and fullness cues, individuals can develop a greater awareness of their body's needs and preferences.
- **Reduced Emotional Eating:** Decreased Emotional Eating: Intuitive eating offers

substitute methods for managing emotions, which results in a decrease in emotional eating habits.

- **Greater Satisfaction with Eating:** By savoring food and eating mindfully, individuals can experience greater satisfaction and enjoyment from their eating experiences.
- **Enhanced Psychological Well-Being:** Intuitive eating is associated with improved self-esteem, body image, and overall psychological well-being.

3. How to Practice Intuitive Eating:

- **Check-In with Your Hunger:** Throughout the day, pause to check in with your body and assess your hunger levels. Eat when you feel physically hungry and stop when you feel satisfied, aiming for a comfortable level of fullness.
- **Eat Mindfully:** Slow down and savor your meals, paying attention to the flavors, textures, and sensations of eating. Minimize distractions and focus on the experience of nourishing your body.
- **Give Yourself Permission to Eat:** Allow yourself to enjoy a variety of foods without judgment or restriction. Honor your cravings and choose foods that satisfy both your physical and emotional hunger.

- **Practice Self-Compassion:** Be gentle and compassionate with yourself as you navigate the journey of intuitive eating. Acknowledge that progress may not always be linear, and give yourself grace during challenging moments.
- **Seek Support:** Surround yourself with supportive friends, family members, or healthcare professionals who understand and respect your intuitive eating journey. Share your experiences, celebrate victories, and seek guidance when needed.

Intuitive eating is a holistic approach to eating that prioritizes self-care, body acceptance, and mindful eating practices. By rejecting diet culture and embracing intuitive eating principles, individuals can foster a healthier relationship with food, enhance their well-being, and cultivate a greater sense of peace and balance in their lives.

- **Mindful Eating Techniques**

Mindful eating is a practice that encourages individuals to bring awareness and attention to their eating experiences, focusing on the present moment without judgment or distraction. By cultivating mindfulness during meals, individuals can develop a deeper connection to their food, body, and emotions, leading to improved eating habits and overall well-being.

1. Cultivating Awareness:

- **Engage the Senses:** Examine the look, smell, and texture of your food for a moment before you consume. Take note of the hues, forms, and designs present on your dish. Take a deep breath in the aroma and enjoy the flavours and scents that emerge. Feel the texture and temperature of your food by running your fingertips over its surface.
- **Check-In with Hunger and Fullness:** Before you eat, take a moment to observe your body and gauge how hungry you are. Measure your level of hunger on a scale of 1 to 10, where 10 represents an uncomfortable full state and 1 represents acute hunger. Throughout the meal, periodically check in with your fullness levels to gauge when you've had enough to eat.

2. Eating Mindfully:

- **Slow Down:** Eat at a relaxed pace, taking the time to chew each bite thoroughly and savor the flavors. Put down your utensils between bites and take a moment to fully experience the taste and texture of your food. Eating slowly allows your body to register feelings of fullness more accurately and promotes better digestion.

- **Focus on Each Bite:** Direct your attention to the sensations of eating, focusing on the flavors, textures, and sensations in your mouth. Notice the subtle changes in taste and texture as you chew your food. Pay attention to the way the food feels against your tongue and the movements of your jaw and throat as you swallow.

- **Be Present:** Practice being fully present with your meal, letting go of distractions and multitasking. Turn off electronic devices, step away from work or other activities, and create a calm and inviting environment for eating. Engage in conversation, if dining with others, but try to maintain awareness of your eating experience throughout the meal.

3. Cultivating Gratitude and Appreciation:

- **Express Gratitude:** Take a moment before eating to express gratitude for the nourishment and sustenance provided by your food. Reflect on the journey of your food from farm to table, acknowledging the efforts of those involved in its production, preparation, and distribution. Cultivating gratitude can enhance the enjoyment and meaning of your eating experiences.

- **Appreciate the Source:** Consider the origins of your food and the natural processes that brought it to your plate. Reflect on the sun, soil, water, and labor that contributed to the growth and cultivation of your food. Connect with the interconnectedness of all living beings and express reverence for the gifts of the earth.

4. Responding to Cravings and Emotions:

- **Observe Cravings Without Judgment:** When cravings arise, observe them with curiosity and compassion, without rushing to fulfill them or suppressing them. Notice the thoughts, sensations, and emotions that accompany your cravings, and explore the underlying reasons behind them. Practice self-compassion and non-judgment as you navigate your relationship with food.
- **Pause Before Eating Emotionally:** If you find yourself turning to food in response to emotions, take a pause before eating and inquire into the emotional triggers behind your cravings. Ask yourself what you're truly hungry for—whether it's comfort, connection, or reassurance—and explore alternative ways of meeting those needs without resorting to food.

5. Reflecting on Satisfaction:

- **Reflect on Satisfaction:** After finishing your meal, take a moment to reflect on your level of satisfaction and contentment. Notice how your body feels physically and emotionally after eating. Pay attention to any feelings of comfort, nourishment, or pleasure that arise from the eating experience. Reflect on the ways in which your food choices support your well-being and vitality.
- **Learn from Experience:** Use each eating experience as an opportunity for learning and growth. Notice patterns, preferences, and reactions to different foods, and adjust your choices accordingly. Cultivate self-awareness and insight into your eating habits, recognizing the interconnectedness between food, mood, and overall health.

Mindful eating techniques involve bringing awareness, attention, and intention to the eating experience, fostering a deeper connection to food, body, and emotions. By practicing mindfulness during meals, individuals can develop healthier eating habits, improve digestion, and enhance their overall well-being. Mindful eating is not about perfection but rather about cultivating presence and compassion in each moment of nourishment.

Developing a Healthy Relationship with Food

Developing a healthy relationship with food is essential for overall well-being, as it influences not only physical health but also emotional and psychological wellness. A healthy relationship with food involves adopting balanced eating habits, cultivating mindfulness and self-awareness, and fostering a positive attitude toward food and body image. Here's a detailed exploration of strategies for developing a healthy relationship with food:

1. Understanding Nutritional Needs:

- **Learn About Nutrition:** Educate yourself about the basic principles of nutrition, including the importance of macronutrients (carbohydrates, proteins, and fats), micronutrients (vitamins and minerals), and hydration. Understand how different nutrients support bodily functions, energy levels, and overall health.
- **Practice Balanced Eating:** Strive to incorporate a variety of nutrient-dense foods into your diet, including fruits, vegetables, whole grains, lean proteins, and healthy fats.

Aim for a balanced plate at each meal, with a combination of carbohydrates, proteins, and fats to support sustained energy and satiety.

2. Cultivating Mindful Eating Habits:

- **Eat with Awareness:** Practice mindfulness during meals by paying attention to the sensory experience of eating, including the flavors, textures, and aromas of your food. Slow down and savor each bite, chewing thoroughly and allowing yourself to fully experience the taste and satisfaction of eating.
- **Tune into Hunger and Fullness:** Listen to your body's hunger and fullness cues to guide your eating decisions. Eat when you're physically hungry and stop when you're comfortably satisfied, aiming for a balance between nourishment and enjoyment.

3. Building Positive Eating Behaviors:

- **Avoid Restrictive Diets:** Steer clear of restrictive diets or fad eating plans that promote extreme food rules or eliminate entire food groups. Instead, focus on adopting a flexible and sustainable approach to eating that emphasizes balance, moderation, and variety.

- **Practice Gentle Nutrition:** Prioritize foods that nourish your body and support your overall health, while also allowing room for enjoyment and flexibility. Aim for a pattern of eating that feels satisfying, enjoyable, and sustainable in the long term.

4. Cultivating a Healthy Body Image:

- **Practice Self-Compassion:** Treat yourself with kindness and compassion, recognizing that your worth is not determined by your body size or appearance. Challenge negative self-talk and cultivate a positive and accepting attitude toward yourself, regardless of your shape or weight.
- **Focus on Health, Not Weight:** Shift your focus away from weight loss and instead prioritize health-promoting behaviors such as regular physical activity, adequate sleep, stress management, and nourishing your body with wholesome foods.

5. Nurturing Emotional Wellness:

- **Explore Emotional Triggers:** Identify emotional triggers that may influence your eating habits, such as stress, boredom, loneliness, or negative emotions. Develop alternative coping strategies for managing emotions without turning to food, such as journaling, mindfulness meditation, deep breathing exercises, or engaging in creative activities.

- **Seek Help When Needed**: If you're having trouble with emotional eating, disordered eating patterns, or negative body image, get help and direction from friends, family, or mental health specialists. Keep in mind that you don't have to travel this path alone and that asking for assistance is a show of courage and resiliency.

6. Promoting Body Respect and Acceptance:

- **Celebrate Your Body:** Focus on the functionality and resilience of your body, appreciating its ability to move, heal, and adapt to life's challenges. Engage in activities that make you feel strong, empowered, and connected to your body, whether it's yoga, dance, walking in nature, or engaging in hobbies you enjoy.
- **Challenge Unrealistic Standards:** Recognize the harmful impact of societal beauty standards and unrealistic portrayals of bodies in the media. Surround yourself with diverse representations of beauty and challenge narrow definitions of attractiveness that prioritize thinness or perfection.

7. Embracing Enjoyable and Pleasurable Eating Experiences:

- **Cultivate Joyful Eating:** Infuse your eating experiences with joy, pleasure, and celebration. Explore new foods, flavors, and culinary traditions that excite your senses and awaken your palate. Share meals with loved ones, savoring the connection and camaraderie that comes with shared dining experiences.
- **Release Guilt and Shame:** Let go of feelings of guilt or shame associated with food choices or eating behaviors. Remember that food is meant to be enjoyed and nourishing, and that a single meal or snack does not define your worth or your health journey.

Developing a healthy relationship with food involves adopting balanced eating habits, cultivating mindfulness and self-awareness, fostering a positive attitude toward food and body image, and prioritizing emotional wellness and self-care. By embracing a holistic approach to eating and nurturing a compassionate and accepting relationship with oneself, individuals can foster long-term well-being and enjoyment in their relationship with food.

Chapter 4

Building a Support System

- ## Seeking Professional Help

Seeking professional help is a crucial step for individuals who are struggling with disordered eating patterns, unhealthy relationships with food, or negative body image. Professional support can provide guidance, validation, and practical strategies for navigating the complexities of eating disorders and promoting recovery.

1. Recognizing the Need for Professional Help:

- **Identifying Signs and Symptoms:** Recognize the signs and symptoms of disordered eating behaviors, including restrictive eating, binge eating, purging, excessive exercise, preoccupation with food or body weight, and distorted body image. Be aware of changes in eating habits, mood, and behavior that may indicate a need for professional intervention.
- **Assessing Impact on Daily Life:** Consider how your relationship with food and body image is affecting your physical health, emotional well-being, relationships, and overall quality of life. Reflect on the extent to which food and body-related concerns are

interfering with your ability to function effectively and engage in meaningful activities.

2. Finding the Right Professional Support:

- **Seeking Qualified Providers:** Look for healthcare professionals who specialize in the treatment of eating disorders, disordered eating, or body image concerns. This may include registered dietitians, therapists, psychologists, psychiatrists, medical doctors, or other specialists with expertise in eating disorder treatment and recovery.
- **Considering Treatment Settings:** Explore different treatment settings and modalities based on your individual needs and preferences. Options may include outpatient therapy, intensive outpatient programs (IOPs), partial hospitalization programs (PHPs), residential treatment centers, or inpatient hospitalization for more severe cases.
- **Seeking Culturally Competent Care:** Consider seeking care from professionals who are culturally competent and sensitive to issues of diversity, identity, and intersectionality. Look for providers who understand the unique cultural, social, and familial factors that may influence your relationship with food and body image.

3. Building a Support Network:

- **Engaging Family and Friends:** Involve supportive family members, friends, or loved ones in your recovery journey. Seek their understanding, encouragement, and validation as you navigate the challenges of seeking professional help and making changes to your eating behaviors and lifestyle.
- **Connecting with Peer Support:** Consider joining support groups, online communities, or peer-led recovery programs for individuals with similar experiences. Peer support offers tools and strategies for overcoming obstacles as well as a feeling of empathy, shared understanding, and companionship.

4. Making the Most of Therapy and Treatment:

- **Establishing Trust and Rapport:** Build a trusting and collaborative relationship with your treatment providers based on open communication, mutual respect, and shared goals. Feel free to ask questions, express concerns, and provide feedback about your treatment experience.
- **Setting Realistic Goals:** Work with your treatment team to set realistic and achievable

goals for your recovery journey. Break down larger goals into smaller, manageable steps, and celebrate progress and milestones along the way.

- **Exploring Evidence-Based Therapies:** Consider evidence-based therapies for eating disorders, such as cognitive-behavioral therapy (CBT), dialectical behavior therapy (DBT), acceptance and commitment therapy (ACT), interpersonal therapy (IPT), or family-based therapy (FBT). These therapies address underlying psychological, emotional, and relational factors contributing to disordered eating behaviors.

5. Navigating Challenges and Setbacks:

- **Coping with Resistance and Ambivalence:** Recognize that ambivalence and resistance to change are normal parts of the recovery process. Be patient and compassionate with yourself as you navigate the ups and downs of recovery, and acknowledge that setbacks are opportunities for learning and growth.
- **Addressing Co-occurring Conditions:** Address any co-occurring mental health conditions, such as anxiety, depression, trauma, or substance use disorders, that may be contributing to your eating disorder symptoms. Seek integrated treatment

approaches that address both eating disorder symptoms and underlying mental health issues.

6. Advocating for Your Needs:

- **Asserting Your Rights:** Advocate for your rights as a patient, including the right to receive informed consent, the right to confidentiality and privacy, and the right to participate in treatment decisions that affect your care. Assert your boundaries and preferences regarding treatment approaches, therapeutic techniques, and medication options.
- **Seeking Second Opinions:** Don't hesitate to seek second opinions or explore alternative treatment options if you feel that your current treatment plan is not meeting your needs or aligning with your recovery goals. Your well-being is paramount, and it's important to find a treatment approach that feels empowering and supportive for you.

Seeking professional help for issues related to food and body image is an important step toward healing, recovery, and empowerment. By reaching out to qualified providers, building a supportive network, engaging in evidence-based therapies, and advocating for your needs, you can embark on a journey of self-discovery, growth, and transformation toward a healthier and more fulfilling relationship with food and your body.

- **Finding Support Groups**

Finding support groups can be a very helpful tool for people who are dealing with eating disorders, body image problems, and food-related problems. Support groups offer a safe and empathetic space for individuals to share their experiences, receive validation, gain insights, and access practical strategies for coping with challenges and fostering recovery.

1. Understanding Support Groups:

- **Peer-Led Communities:** Support groups are typically peer-led communities of individuals who share common experiences, challenges, or concerns related to food, body image, disordered eating, or eating disorders. These groups provide a non-judgmental and supportive environment for sharing stories, offering encouragement, and seeking guidance from others who understand firsthand what you're going through.
- **Varied Formats:** Support groups may take various formats, including in-person meetings, virtual gatherings, online forums,

chat rooms, or social media groups. Some groups may be facilitated by mental health professionals, while others may be self-directed or led by individuals in recovery.

2. Finding Support Groups:

- **Online Resources:** Explore online resources and directories to find support groups that align with your specific needs and preferences. Websites such as the National Eating Disorders Association (NEDA), Eating Disorder Hope, and Psychology Today offer searchable databases of support groups, treatment providers, and community resources.
- **Mental Health Agencies**: Find out about support groups for eating disorders or body image issues by getting in touch with local clinics, hospitals, treatment facilities, or mental health organisations. As part of their services, a lot of organisations provide peer support groups, courses, and group treatment programmes.
- **Professional Referrals:** Ask your healthcare provider, therapist, or registered dietitian for recommendations for support groups in your community. They may be able to provide referrals to reputable organizations or groups that specialize in eating disorder recovery and support.

3. Evaluating Support Groups:

- **Mission and Values:** Consider the mission, values, and guiding principles of the support group to ensure that they align with your personal beliefs and goals for recovery. Look for groups that prioritize inclusivity, empathy, respect, and empowerment, and that promote a non-judgmental and supportive atmosphere for all members.
- **Accessibility and Inclusivity:** Evaluate the accessibility and inclusivity of the support group in terms of location, meeting times, language, cultural sensitivity, and accommodations for individuals with diverse needs or identities. Choose groups that prioritize accessibility and strive to create a welcoming and inclusive environment for all participants.

4. Participating in Support Groups:

- **Active Participation:** Actively engage in group discussions, sharing your experiences, insights, challenges, and successes with other members. Be open to listening to others' perspectives and offering support and encouragement in return.
- **Respect and Confidentiality:** Respect the confidentiality and privacy of group members by refraining from sharing

personal information or stories outside of the group setting. Create a safe and trusting space where members feel comfortable expressing themselves without fear of judgment or breach of confidentiality.

- **Setting Boundaries:** Set boundaries around topics of discussion and personal sharing that feel comfortable and appropriate for you. It's okay to participate at your own pace and to opt out of discussions or activities that feel triggering or overwhelming.

5. Benefits of Support Groups:

- **Validation and Understanding:** Support groups provide validation and understanding from individuals who share similar experiences and challenges related to food, body image, and eating disorders. Sharing stories and insights with others who "get it" can foster a sense of connection, belonging, and validation.
- **Practical Strategies:** Support groups offer practical strategies, coping skills, and recovery tools for managing challenges, coping with triggers, and fostering positive changes in eating behaviors and body image. Members can learn from each other's experiences and share insights and resources for self-care and healing.

- **Emotional Support:** Support groups offer emotional support and empathy during difficult times, providing a source of comfort, encouragement, and solidarity for individuals navigating the ups and downs of recovery. Knowing that you're not alone in your journey can provide a sense of hope and resilience.

6. Navigating Challenges:

- **Managing Triggers:** Be mindful of potential triggers or emotional reactions that may arise during group discussions. Practice self-care techniques such as deep breathing, grounding exercises, or mindfulness meditation to help regulate emotions and manage triggers effectively.
- **Seeking Professional Help:** While support groups can be a valuable complement to professional treatment, they may not be a substitute for individual therapy, medical care, or nutritional counseling. If you're struggling with severe or persistent symptoms, consider seeking guidance from a mental health professional or healthcare provider for personalized support and treatment.

Finding support groups can be a valuable source of connection, validation, and encouragement for individuals struggling with issues related to food, body image, and eating disorders. By actively participating in supportive communities, individuals can gain insights, learn coping strategies, and foster resilience on their journey toward healing and recovery.

- **Enlisting Friends and Family Support**

Enlisting the support of friends and family is a crucial aspect of recovery for individuals struggling with issues related to food, body image, and eating disorders. Friends and family members can play a pivotal role in providing emotional support, encouragement, and practical assistance throughout the recovery journey. Here's an in-depth analysis of getting help from friends and family:

1. Educating Loved Ones:

- **Raise Awareness:** Educate friends and family members about eating disorders, disordered eating behaviors, and body image concerns. Help them understand the complexities of these issues, including the psychological, emotional, and physical factors involved.

- **Provide Resources:** Give friends and family access to reliable websites, books, articles, and resources regarding eating disorders and recovery. Urge them to read up on eating disorder symptoms and signs as well as ways that they may help you on your road to recovery.

2. Communicating Openly and Honestly:

- **Open Dialogue:** Foster open and honest communication with friends and family members about your struggles, challenges, and goals for recovery. Share your feelings, thoughts, and concerns openly, and encourage loved ones to do the same.
- **Express Needs and Boundaries:** Clearly communicate your needs, boundaries, and preferences for support to friends and family members. Let them know how they can best support you during difficult times and what actions or comments may be triggering or unhelpful.

3. Setting Realistic Expectations:

- **Manage Expectations:** Help friends and family members understand that recovery from an eating disorder or body image concerns is a complex and nonlinear process that takes time, patience, and persistence.

Set realistic expectations for the recovery journey and emphasize the importance of progress over perfection.

- **Celebrate Small Victories:** Celebrate little accomplishments and turning points in your journey, including overcoming a fear of certain foods, taking care of yourself, or getting help from a professional. No matter how small the steps you take to progress may seem, encourage friends and family to acknowledge and appreciate your accomplishments.

4. Providing Emotional Support:

- **Offer Empathy and Understanding:** Provide empathy, understanding, and non-judgmental support by your loved one as you navigate the challenges of recovery. They should listen actively, validate your feelings, and offer reassurance that you're not alone in your struggles.
- **Be Present and Available:** They should be present and available for you during difficult moments or times of crisis. Offer a listening ear, a shoulder to lean on, or a comforting presence without trying to fix or solve your problems.

5. Encouraging Healthy Coping Strategies:

- **Promote Self-Care:** Encourage you to prioritize self-care practices such as relaxation techniques, mindfulness meditation, creative expression, or spending time in nature. Help you identify healthy coping strategies that promote emotional well-being and stress management.
- **Model Healthy Behaviors:** They should lead by example by modeling healthy behaviors and attitudes toward food, body image, and self-care. Demonstrate balance, moderation, and flexibility in their own eating habits and lifestyle choices.

6. Seeking Support for Caregivers:

- **Self-Care for Caregivers:** Encourage friends and family members to prioritize their own self-care and well-being as caregivers. Remind them that supporting a loved one with an eating disorder can be emotionally taxing and that they also need to take care of themselves in order to provide effective support.
- **Accessing Support Networks:** Encourage caregivers to seek support from other caregivers, support groups, or mental health professionals to share experiences, gain

insights, and receive validation and encouragement in their caregiving role.

8. Navigating Challenges and Setbacks:

- **Managing Frustration and Helplessness:** Acknowledge and validate feelings of frustration, helplessness, or uncertainty that may arise as a caregiver supporting a loved one with an eating disorder. Practice self-compassion and seek support from others who understand your experiences.
- **Seeking Professional Guidance:** Encourage your loved one to seek professional guidance and support from therapists, registered dietitians, medical doctors, or other healthcare providers specializing in eating disorder treatment and recovery. Collaborate with treatment providers to develop a comprehensive and individualized treatment plan that addresses your loved one's unique needs and challenges.

Enlisting the support of friends and family is an essential component of recovery for individuals struggling with eating disorders, disordered eating behaviors, or body image concerns. By fostering open communication, setting realistic expectations, providing emotional support, encouraging healthy coping strategies, collaborating in treatment and recovery, and seeking support for caregivers, friends and family members can play a valuable role in supporting their loved one's journey toward healing

Chapter 5

Coping Strategies

• Stress Management Techniques

Stress management techniques are essential tools for coping with the demands and pressures of daily life, promoting relaxation, and maintaining overall well-being. Effective stress management strategies can help reduce the negative effects of stress on both physical and mental health, improve resilience, and enhance quality of life. Below are some stress management techniques:

1. Mindfulness and Meditation:

- **Mindfulness Practice:** Mindfulness involves bringing non-judgmental awareness to the present moment, observing thoughts, emotions, and sensations without reacting to them. Mindfulness techniques, such as focused breathing, body scans, or mindful walking, can help calm the mind and promote relaxation.
- **Meditation:** Meditation practices, such as mindfulness meditation, loving-kindness meditation, or body scan meditation, can help reduce stress, increase self-awareness, and cultivate a sense of inner peace and tranquility. Regular meditation practice can

train the mind to become more resilient in the face of stressors.

2. Deep Breathing Exercises:

- **Diaphragmatic Breathing:** Deep breathing exercises, also known as diaphragmatic or belly breathing, involve taking slow, deep breaths that engage the diaphragm and activate the body's relaxation response. Deep breathing can help lower stress hormones, reduce muscle tension, and promote feelings of calm and relaxation.
- **Box Breathing:** Box breathing is a technique that involves inhaling for a count of four, holding the breath for a count of four, exhaling for a count of four, and holding the breath again for a count of four, creating a square or box pattern. Box breathing can help regulate the nervous system and induce a state of calmness.

3. Progressive Muscle Relaxation (PMR):

- **Muscle Relaxation:** Progressive muscle relaxation is a technique that involves systematically tensing and relaxing different muscle groups in the body, starting from the toes and working your way up to the head. PMR helps release physical tension, reduce muscle stiffness, and promote a sense of relaxation and well-being.

4. Exercise and Physical Activity:

- **Regular Exercise:** Engaging in regular physical activity, such as walking, jogging, swimming, yoga, or dancing, can help reduce stress levels, improve mood, and boost overall resilience to stress. Exercise releases endorphins, the body's natural feel-good chemicals, which can help counteract the negative effects of stress.
- **Outdoor Activities:** Spending time in nature and engaging in outdoor activities, such as hiking, gardening, or simply taking a stroll in a park, can have a calming effect on the mind and body. Nature has been shown to promote relaxation, reduce anxiety, and improve overall well-being.

5. Healthy Lifestyle Habits:

- **Balanced Nutrition:** Eating a balanced diet rich in fruits, vegetables, whole grains, lean proteins, and healthy fats can provide the body with essential nutrients and energy needed to cope with stress. Avoid excessive consumption of caffeine, sugar, and processed foods, which can exacerbate stress and anxiety.

- **Adequate Sleep:** Prioritize getting sufficient sleep each night, aiming for seven to nine hours of quality sleep for most adults. Poor sleep can increase stress levels, impair cognitive function, and weaken the body's ability to cope with stressors. Establish a relaxing bedtime routine and create a comfortable sleep environment to promote restful sleep.
- **Limiting Alcohol and Substance Use:** Limit alcohol consumption and avoid recreational drugs or substances as a means of coping with stress. Alcohol and drugs may provide temporary relief from stress but can ultimately aggravate anxiety, depression, and other mental health issues.

6. Time Management and Prioritization:

- **Setting Priorities:** Identify tasks and responsibilities that are most important and prioritize them accordingly. Break down larger tasks into smaller, manageable steps and focus on completing one task at a time to avoid feeling overwhelmed.
- **Effective Planning:** Use organizational tools, such as calendars, to-do lists, or digital apps, to plan and schedule activities, appointments, and deadlines. Allocate time for work, relaxation, social activities, and

self-care to maintain a healthy balance in your life.

7. Seeking Social Support:

- **Connecting with Others:** Reach out to friends, family members, or support networks for emotional support and companionship during times of stress. Sharing experiences, expressing feelings, and receiving encouragement from others can help alleviate feelings of isolation and loneliness.
- **Joining Support Groups:** Consider joining support groups or community organizations that provide a safe and empathetic space for individuals to share their experiences, gain insights, and access practical strategies for coping with stress and adversity.

8. Practicing Self-Care:

- **Self-Compassion:** Treat yourself with kindness, compassion, and understanding during times of stress. Practice self-compassion by acknowledging your efforts and strengths, accepting imperfections, and being gentle with yourself during difficult moments.
- **Engaging in Activities You Enjoy:** Make time for activities and hobbies that bring you

joy, fulfillment, and relaxation. Engage in creative pursuits, hobbies, or leisure activities that nourish your spirit and help you recharge physically, mentally, and emotionally.

Stress management techniques encompass a variety of strategies aimed at promoting relaxation, reducing tension, and enhancing resilience in the face of stressors. By incorporating mindfulness practices, deep breathing exercises, progressive muscle relaxation, regular exercise, healthy lifestyle habits, effective time management, social support, and self-care into your daily routine, you can develop a comprehensive toolkit for managing stress and improving overall well-being. Experiment with different techniques to find what works best for you, and remember that consistency and practice are key to experiencing the benefits of stress management strategies over time.

- **Healthy Distractions**

Healthy distractions are activities or practices that help individuals shift their focus away from stressors, worries, or negative thoughts, promoting relaxation, enjoyment, and a sense of well-being. Engaging in healthy distractions can provide a temporary reprieve from challenging emotions or situations, allowing individuals to recharge mentally and emotionally. Examples of healthy distractions:

1. Creative Pursuits:

- **Artistic Expression:** Engaging in creative activities such as drawing, painting, sculpting, or crafting can serve as a therapeutic outlet for self-expression and stress relief. Creative pursuits allow individuals to tap into their imagination, explore emotions, and channel their energy into meaningful projects.
- **Writing and Journaling:** Writing can be a powerful tool for processing emotions, gaining clarity, and capturing thoughts and experiences. Journaling allows individuals to express themselves freely, document their journey, and gain insights into patterns, triggers, and coping strategies.

2. Physical Activities:

- **Exercise:** Physical activity is known to release endorphins, the body's natural feel-good chemicals, which can help alleviate stress, anxiety, and depression. Engage in activities such as walking, jogging, cycling, swimming, or dancing to boost mood, increase energy levels, and improve overall well-being.

- **Yoga and Tai Chi:** Mind-body practices such as yoga and tai chi combine gentle movements with focused breathing and mindfulness techniques to promote relaxation, flexibility, and inner peace. These practices can help reduce muscle tension, calm the mind, and enhance mind-body awareness.

3. Nature and Outdoor Activities:

- **Spending Time in Nature:** Connecting with nature can have a grounding and rejuvenating effect on the mind and body. Spend time outdoors, whether it's going for a nature walk, hiking in the mountains, or simply enjoying the beauty of a park or garden. Nature provides a soothing backdrop for relaxation and reflection.
- **Gardening:** Gardening offers a hands-on way to connect with nature, nurture living plants, and engage in mindful activities such as planting, weeding, and harvesting. Gardening can be a therapeutic and rewarding hobby that fosters a sense of connection to the natural world.

4. Social Connections:

- **Connecting with Loved Ones:** Spending time with friends, family members, or supportive peers can provide comfort, companionship, and a sense of belonging. Engage in meaningful conversations, share laughter and stories, and strengthen relationships with loved ones.

- **Joining Clubs or Groups:** Joining clubs, community organizations, or hobby groups allows individuals to pursue shared interests, meet like-minded individuals, and engage in enjoyable activities together. Participating in group activities fosters a sense of camaraderie and social connection.

5. Learning and Intellectual Stimulation:

- **Reading:** Reading can transport individuals to different worlds, stimulate imagination, and provide an escape from daily stressors. Whether it's fiction, non-fiction, poetry, or literature, reading offers a form of mental stimulation and relaxation.
- **Learning New Skills:** Engaging in learning activities or acquiring new skills can be both intellectually stimulating and personally fulfilling. Whether it's learning a musical instrument, mastering a new language, or exploring a new hobby, the process of learning fosters growth, curiosity, and self-discovery.

6. Mindfulness and Relaxation Practices:

- **Mindfulness Meditation:** Mindfulness meditation involves paying attention to the present moment with openness, curiosity, and acceptance. Practicing mindfulness meditation can help individuals cultivate awareness, reduce rumination, and develop a sense of calm amidst life's challenges.

7. Volunteer Work and Acts of Kindness:

- **Giving Back:** Engaging in volunteer work or acts of kindness can provide a sense of purpose, fulfillment, and connection to others. Whether it's volunteering at a local charity, participating in community service projects, or helping a neighbor in need, giving back to others can be deeply rewarding.

8. Limiting Screen Time and Digital Detox:

- **Unplugging from Technology:** Take breaks from electronic devices and screens to reduce exposure to digital stimuli and create space for mindfulness and reflection. Engage in activities that don't involve screens, such as spending time outdoors, engaging in hobbies, or enjoying face-to-face interactions with others.

Healthy distractions offer individuals a variety of ways to temporarily shift their focus away from stressors, worries, or negative emotions, promoting relaxation, enjoyment, and a sense of well-being. By incorporating creative pursuits, physical activities, nature experiences, social connections, learning opportunities, mindfulness practices, acts of kindness, and screen-free time into their daily lives, individuals can cultivate resilience, balance, and inner peace in the face of life's challenges. Experiment with different healthy distractions to discover what resonates best with you and prioritize self-care as an essential part of your well-being routine.

- **Relaxation and Meditation**

Relaxation and meditation are powerful practices that promote physical, mental, and emotional well-being by inducing a state of calm, reducing stress, and enhancing overall resilience. Both relaxation and meditation techniques can be integrated into daily life to cultivate a greater sense of peace, clarity, and inner harmony.

1. Understanding Relaxation:

- **Physical Relaxation:** Relaxation involves intentionally releasing tension and stress from the body, allowing muscles to unwind and promoting a sense of physical ease and comfort. Physical relaxation techniques target areas of tension, such as the neck, shoulders, back, and jaw, to promote relaxation throughout the body.

- **Mental Relaxation:** Mental relaxation focuses on quieting the mind, calming racing thoughts, and reducing mental chatter and distractions. Mental relaxation techniques help individuals cultivate a sense of inner calm, clarity, and mindfulness amidst the busyness of daily life.

2. Techniques for Relaxation:

- **Deep Breathing Exercises:** Deep breathing techniques, such as diaphragmatic breathing or belly breathing, involve taking slow, deep breaths that engage the diaphragm and activate the body's relaxation response. Deep breathing can help reduce stress hormones, lower blood pressure, and promote a sense of calm and relaxation.
- **Progressive Muscle Relaxation (PMR):** Progressive muscle relaxation is a technique that involves systematically tensing and relaxing different muscle groups in the body, starting from the toes and working your way up to the head. PMR helps release physical tension, reduce muscle stiffness, and promote relaxation throughout the body.

- **Visualization and Guided Imagery:** Visualization techniques involve mentally picturing calming scenes, images, or scenarios that evoke feelings of relaxation and tranquility. Guided imagery scripts or recordings can lead individuals through visualizations of peaceful settings, such as a beach, forest, or meadow, to promote relaxation and stress relief.
- **Body Scan Meditation:** Body scan meditation involves systematically directing attention to different parts of the body, starting from the toes and moving upward, while noticing sensations, tension, or areas of discomfort. Body scan meditation promotes body awareness, relaxation, and mindfulness of physical sensations.

3. Understanding Meditation:

- **Mindfulness Meditation:** Mindfulness meditation involves paying non-judgmental attention to the present moment, observing thoughts, emotions, and sensations as they arise without attachment or reactivity. Mindfulness meditation cultivates awareness, acceptance, and equanimity, allowing individuals to develop a deeper understanding of their inner experience.
- **Focused Attention Meditation:** Focused attention meditation involves directing

attention to a single point of focus, such as the breath, a mantra, or a visual object, while gently redirecting the mind whenever it wanders. Focused attention meditation enhances concentration, mental clarity, and cognitive control.

- **Loving-Kindness Meditation:** Loving-kindness meditation involves cultivating feelings of compassion, kindness, and goodwill toward oneself and others through the repetition of phrases or intentions. Loving-kindness meditation fosters a sense of connection, empathy, and emotional resilience, promoting positive relationships and well-being.

4. Benefits of Relaxation and Meditation:

- **Stress Reduction:** Both relaxation and meditation techniques are effective tools for reducing stress, lowering cortisol levels, and promoting relaxation of the body and mind. Regular practice can help individuals cope with daily stressors more effectively and build resilience to future challenges.
- **Improved Mental Health:** Relaxation and meditation practices have been shown to alleviate symptoms of anxiety, depression, and other mood disorders by promoting emotional regulation, enhancing self-

awareness, and fostering a sense of inner peace and well-being.

- **Enhanced Physical Health:** Relaxation and meditation techniques have numerous physical health benefits, including reducing blood pressure, lowering heart rate, improving sleep quality, and boosting immune function. These practices support overall health and vitality by promoting relaxation and balance in the body.
- **Increased Mindfulness and Awareness:** Meditation cultivates mindfulness, the ability to be present and fully engaged in the present moment, without judgment or distraction. Mindfulness enhances awareness of thoughts, emotions, and sensations, allowing individuals to respond to life's challenges with greater clarity and equanimity.

5. Integrating Relaxation and Meditation into Daily Life:

- **Consistent Practice:** Establish a regular practice of relaxation and meditation, integrating these techniques into your daily routine. Set aside dedicated time each day for formal practice, whether it's in the morning, during lunch breaks, or in the evening before bed.

- **Informal Practice:** Incorporate informal mindfulness practices into daily activities, such as mindful eating, mindful walking, or mindful listening. Bring mindful awareness to everyday experiences, noticing sensations, thoughts, and emotions as they arise throughout the day.
- **Flexibility and Adaptability:** Explore different relaxation and meditation techniques to find what resonates best with you. Be open to experimenting with different approaches, styles, and durations of practice to discover what feels most supportive and sustainable for your unique needs and preferences.
- **Patience and Compassion:** Approach relaxation and meditation with an attitude of patience, curiosity, and self-compassion. Recognize that meditation is a skill that develops over time and that each moment of practice is an opportunity for learning, growth, and self-discovery.

Relaxation and meditation are invaluable practices for promoting physical, mental, and emotional well-being, cultivating mindfulness, and enhancing overall quality of life. By incorporating relaxation and meditation techniques into daily life and nurturing a consistent practice, individuals can experience greater calm, clarity, and resilience in the face of life's challenges. Experiment with different techniques, remain open to the present moment, and cultivate a spirit of curiosity and compassion on your journey of relaxation and meditation.

73

Chapter 6

Developing Healthy Habits

- ## Meal Planning and Preparation

Meal planning and preparation involve the thoughtful selection of nutritious foods, organization of meals, and cooking of recipes to support health, well-being, and dietary goals. By taking a proactive approach to meal planning and preparation, individuals can save time, reduce stress, and make healthier food choices.

1. Importance of Meal Planning:

- **Nutritional Adequacy:** Meal planning ensures that individuals consume a balanced diet that meets their nutritional needs, including essential nutrients such as vitamins, minerals, protein, carbohydrates, and healthy fats.
- **Health Goals:** Meal planning can help individuals achieve specific health goals, such as weight management, improved energy levels, better digestion, or the prevention and management of chronic diseases like diabetes or heart disease.
- **Budget-Friendly:** Planning meals in advance allows individuals to make cost-effective choices, reduce food waste, and

stick to a budget by buying ingredients in bulk, taking advantage of sales, and avoiding impulse purchases.

2. Steps for Effective Meal Planning:

- **Set Goals and Priorities:** Define your health and nutrition goals, such as increasing vegetable intake, reducing sugar consumption, or cooking more meals at home. Consider dietary preferences, food allergies, and cultural or religious considerations when planning meals.
- **Create a Menu:** Design a weekly or monthly menu that includes a variety of nutrient-dense foods from different food groups, such as fruits, vegetables, whole grains, lean proteins, and healthy fats. Incorporate a mix of colors, flavors, and textures to keep meals interesting and satisfying.
- **Consider Convenience:** Choose recipes and meal options that are simple, convenient, and easy to prepare, especially on busy days. Look for recipes that require minimal ingredients, preparation time, and cooking skills, or consider batch cooking and meal prepping ahead of time.
- **Use Resources:** Explore cookbooks, recipe websites, food blogs, and meal planning apps for inspiration and ideas. Experiment

with new ingredients, cuisines, and cooking techniques to keep meals exciting and flavorful.

- **Shop Wisely:** Make a grocery list based on your planned meals and ingredients needed. Organize your shopping list by food categories or sections of the grocery store to streamline the shopping process and avoid forgetting essential items.

3. Tips for Efficient Meal Preparation:

- **Batch Cooking:** Set aside time each week to batch cook staple ingredients such as grains, proteins, vegetables, and sauces. Prepare large batches of soups, stews, casseroles, or one-pot meals that can be portioned out and enjoyed throughout the week.
- **Prep Ingredients:** Wash, chop, and pre-portion fruits, vegetables, and herbs in advance to streamline meal preparation. Store prepared ingredients in airtight containers or reusable bags in the refrigerator to maintain freshness and convenience.
- **Invest in Kitchen Tools:** Invest in quality kitchen tools and appliances that make meal preparation more efficient and enjoyable, such as a sharp chef's knife, cutting boards,

vegetable peeler, blender, food processor, or slow cooker.

- **Plan for Leftovers:** Embrace leftovers as a convenient and budget-friendly option for meals. Cook extra portions of meals and store leftovers in meal-sized containers for quick and easy lunches or dinners throughout the week.
- **Practice Safe Food Handling:** Follow food safety guidelines when storing, reheating, and consuming leftovers to prevent foodborne illness. Refrigerate perishable foods promptly, reheat leftovers to the proper temperature, and discard any leftovers that have been stored for too long.

4. Benefits of Meal Planning and Preparation:

- **Save Time:** Meal planning and preparation save time by reducing the need for last-minute trips to the grocery store, deciding what to cook on the spot, and waiting for food delivery or takeout orders.
- **Healthier Choices:** By planning meals in advance, individuals can make healthier choices and avoid relying on processed foods, fast food, or convenience foods that may be high in calories, sodium, sugar, and unhealthy fats.
- **Reduce Stress:** Knowing what to eat and having ingredients readily available can

reduce stress and anxiety around mealtime. Meal planning provides a sense of structure, control, and predictability, especially for individuals with busy schedules or dietary restrictions.
- **Financial Savings:** Meal planning and preparation can help individuals save money by reducing food waste, avoiding impulse purchases, and maximizing the use of pantry staples and leftovers.

5. Flexibility and Adaptability:

- **Be Flexible:** Be flexible and adaptable with your meal planning and preparation approach. Allow for changes in schedule, unexpected events, or dietary preferences, and adjust your meal plan accordingly.
- **Experiment and Explore:** Use meal planning and preparation as an opportunity to experiment with new recipes, ingredients, and cooking techniques. Embrace variety and creativity in your meals to keep them interesting and enjoyable.

6. Involve Family and Friends:

- **Family Involvement:** Involve family members or household members in the meal planning and preparation process. Encourage collaboration, creativity, and

> shared responsibility for mealtime decisions and tasks.
> - **Meal Sharing:** Plan meals and enjoy shared meals with family and friends as a way to foster connection, communication, and social support. Share cooking responsibilities, swap recipes, and enjoy the pleasure of dining together.

Meal planning and preparation are essential practices for promoting health, saving time, reducing stress, and making the most of available resources. By taking a proactive and organized approach to meal planning and preparation, individuals can enjoy nutritious, delicious, and satisfying meals that support their well-being and lifestyle goals. Experiment with different strategies, embrace flexibility, and make mealtime an enjoyable and nourishing part of your daily routine.

- **Balanced Nutrition**

Balanced nutrition is a fundamental aspect of maintaining good health and well-being. It refers to consuming a variety of foods in appropriate proportions to provide the body with the necessary nutrients it needs to function optimally. A balanced diet typically includes a combination of macronutrients (carbohydrates, proteins, and fats), micronutrients (vitamins and minerals), fiber, and adequate hydration.

Here's a detailed overview of each component of balanced nutrition:

1. **Macronutrients**:
   - Carbohydrates: The body uses carbohydrates as its main energy source. Foods include grains, fruits, vegetables, and legumes contain them. Because they are higher in fibre and nutrients than refined grains like white bread and pasta, whole grains like brown rice, quinoa, and oats are recommended.
   - Proteins: Building and mending tissues, producing hormones and enzymes, and bolstering the immune system all depend on proteins. Lean meats, poultry, fish, eggs, dairy products, legumes, nuts, and seeds are all excellent sources of protein.
   - Fats: Proper fats are essential for hormone production, nutrition absorption, and cell structure. They also give you energy and support good skin and hair. Avocados, almonds, seeds, olive oil, fatty fish (such as salmon and mackerel), and flaxseeds are foods high in good fats.

2. **Micronutrients**:
- Vitamins: Vitamins are organic compounds that regulate various bodily functions and processes. They are found in a wide range of foods, including fruits, vegetables, whole grains, dairy products, and meats. Different vitamins play roles in energy metabolism, immune function, bone health, and more.
- Minerals: Minerals are inorganic substances that are necessary for neuron function, muscular contraction, bone health, and fluid equilibrium. Dairy products, leafy greens, nuts, seeds, whole grains, and lean meats are good sources of minerals.

3. Fibre: The body is unable to absorb fibre, a form of carbohydrate that is present in plant-based diets. It helps regulate blood sugar levels, facilitates regular bowel movements, aids in digestion, and may lower the chance of developing certain illnesses including diabetes and heart disease. Fruits, vegetables, whole grains, legumes, nuts, and seeds are all excellent sources of fibre.

3. **Hydration**:
   - Water is essential for various bodily functions, including regulating body temperature, transporting nutrients, flushing out toxins, and lubricating joints. It is crucial to stay adequately hydrated throughout the day by drinking water and consuming water-rich foods like fruits and vegetables.

A balanced diet emphasizes the importance of moderation, variety, and portion control. It involves choosing a wide range of nutrient-dense foods from different food groups to ensure that the body receives all the essential nutrients it needs to thrive. Additionally, incorporating mindful eating habits, such as paying attention to hunger and fullness cues, can help individuals maintain a healthy relationship with food and make informed dietary choices. Overall, balanced nutrition plays a critical role in promoting overall health, supporting growth and development, and reducing the risk of chronic diseases.

- **Regular Exercise**

Regular exercise is a cornerstone of a healthy lifestyle and is essential for maintaining physical and mental well-being. It encompasses a wide range of physical activities that engage the body's muscles, cardiovascular system, and various physiological processes. Incorporating regular exercise into one's routine offers numerous benefits and plays a crucial role in promoting overall health and longevity.

Here's a comprehensive overview of the importance and components of regular exercise:

- **Physical Health Benefits**:
    - **Cardiovascular Health**: Regular exercise helps lower blood pressure and cholesterol, strengthens the heart muscle, and enhances circulation. It lowers the chance of stroke, heart disease, and other cardiovascular disorders.
    - **Weight Management**: Engaging in physical activity helps burn calories and maintain a healthy weight. Combining exercise with a balanced diet is an effective strategy for managing body weight and preventing obesity.
    - **Muscle Strength and Flexibility**: Exercise helps build and maintain muscle mass, strength, and endurance. It also enhances flexibility, agility, and coordination, which are essential for performing daily activities and preventing injuries.

- **Bone Health**: Weight-bearing exercises, such as walking, jogging, and strength training, promote bone density and reduce the risk of osteoporosis and bone fractures, especially in older adults.
- **Improved Immune Function**: Regular moderate-intensity exercise can boost the immune system, reduce the risk of infections, and enhance the body's ability to fight off illness and disease.
- **Mental Health Benefits**:
  - **Stress Reduction**: Exercise stimulates the production of endorphins, neurotransmitters that promote feelings of happiness and well-being. It helps alleviate stress, anxiety, and depression, and improves mood and overall mental outlook.
  - **Enhanced Cognitive Function**: Physical activity has been linked to improved cognitive function, memory, and concentration. It promotes neuroplasticity, the brain's ability to form new connections and adapt to challenges.
  - **Better Sleep Quality**: Regular exercise can improve sleep quality and duration by regulating sleep-wake cycles and promoting relaxation. It

helps individuals fall asleep faster and experience deeper, more restorative sleep.

- **Boosted Self-Esteem and Confidence**: Achieving fitness goals and experiencing improvements in physical strength and endurance can enhance self-esteem, self-confidence, and body image.

- **Social Interaction**: Engaging in outdoor activities, sports teams, or group exercise courses offers chances for community involvement, friendship, and social interaction—all of which improve one's general well-being.

- **Types of Exercise**:
    - **Aerobic Exercise**: Activities like walking, running, cycling, swimming, dancing, and aerobics increase heart rate and breathing rate, improving cardiovascular fitness and endurance.
    - **Strength Training**: Muscle strength, power, and endurance can be increased through resistance training with weights, resistance bands, or your own body weight. They also aid in metabolism and bone health.
    - **Flexibility and Balance Exercises**: Particularly for older persons, stretching, yoga, tai chi, and Pilates

enhance flexibility, balance, and posture while lowering the risk of falls and injuries.

- **Interval Training**: High-intensity interval training (HIIT) alternates between short bursts of intense exercise and brief periods of rest or lower-intensity activity. It enhances cardiovascular fitness, burns calories, and improves metabolic function.

Regular exercise is a critical component of a healthy lifestyle, offering numerous physical, mental, and emotional benefits. Incorporating a variety of activities that address cardiovascular fitness, strength, flexibility, and balance into one's routine can help individuals achieve and maintain optimal health and well-being at every stage of life. Additionally, adopting a consistent exercise regimen and making physical activity a priority can lead to long-term improvements in overall quality of life.

87

Chapter 7

Overcoming Emotional Eating

- ### Understanding Emotions and Food

Understanding the relationship between emotions and food is essential for promoting healthy eating habits and emotional well-being. Many people experience a complex interplay between their emotions and food choices, often turning to food for comfort, stress relief, or as a way to cope with difficult emotions. This phenomenon can have both positive and negative implications for individuals' physical and emotional health.

Here's a detailed exploration of the connection between emotions and food:

1. **Emotional Eating**:
   - **Comfort Eating**: People often turn to food for comfort during times of stress, sadness, loneliness, or boredom. Certain foods, particularly those high in sugar, fat, and salt, may trigger the release of feel-good neurotransmitters like serotonin and temporarily alleviate negative emotions.
   - **Reward Eating**: Food can be used as a reward or a form of self-soothing

after a challenging day or as a way to celebrate achievements and milestones. This behavior can become ingrained as a habitual response to certain emotions or situations.

- **Mindless Eating**: Eating out of boredom or habit without paying attention to hunger cues or nutritional needs can lead to overeating and weight gain. Distractions such as watching television or scrolling through social media can contribute to mindless eating habits.

2. **Food and Mood**:
   - **Nutritional Impact**: Certain nutrients and dietary patterns can influence mood and emotional well-being. For example, foods rich in omega-3 fatty acids, vitamins, minerals, and antioxidants may have antidepressant and mood-stabilizing effects.
   - **Blood Sugar Regulation**: Fluctuations in blood sugar levels can affect mood and energy levels. Consuming high-sugar foods can lead to temporary spikes in blood sugar followed by crashes, resulting in mood swings, irritability, and fatigue.
   - **Gut-Brain Connection**: Emerging research suggests that the gut microbiota play a crucial role in

regulating mood and behavior through the gut-brain axis. A healthy diet rich in fiber, probiotics, and prebiotics can support gut health and promote emotional well-being.

- **Food Allergies and Sensitivities**: Certain individuals may experience mood disturbances and emotional symptoms in response to food allergies, intolerances, or sensitivities. Identifying and eliminating trigger foods can alleviate symptoms and improve overall mood.

3. **Coping Strategies**:
   - **Mindful Eating**: Practicing mindfulness techniques can help individuals become more aware of their eating habits, emotions, and hunger cues. Mindful eating involves paying attention to the sensory experience of eating, savoring each bite, and tuning into feelings of hunger and satiety.
   - **Emotion Regulation**: Developing healthy coping mechanisms for managing emotions, such as stress management techniques, relaxation exercises, journaling, and seeking support from friends, family, or mental health professionals, can

reduce the reliance on food as a primary coping strategy.

- **Creating Healthy Habits**: Cultivating a balanced and varied diet composed of whole foods, fruits, vegetables, lean proteins, whole grains, and healthy fats can support emotional well-being and overall health. Establishing regular meal times, planning nutritious meals and snacks, and practicing portion control can help foster a positive relationship with food.

Understanding the complex interplay between emotions and food is crucial for promoting mindful eating habits, emotional regulation, and overall well-being. By fostering awareness of emotional triggers, developing healthy coping strategies, and cultivating a balanced approach to nutrition, individuals can nurture a positive relationship with food and support their physical, emotional, and mental health goals.

- **Finding Alternative Coping Mechanisms**

Finding alternative coping mechanisms is an essential aspect of emotional resilience and mental health. Coping mechanisms are strategies individuals use to manage stress, anxiety, and other difficult emotions or situations. While some coping mechanisms may be helpful and adaptive, others can be harmful or ineffective in the long term. Therefore, finding alternative coping mechanisms involves identifying healthier, more constructive ways to deal with challenges and emotions. Here's a detailed look at how to find alternative coping mechanisms:

1. Self-awareness:

- **Identify Current Coping Mechanisms:** Start by recognizing the coping mechanisms you currently use. This could include behaviors like avoidance, substance use, overeating, or lashing out.
- **Assess Effectiveness:** Evaluate how well your current coping mechanisms work for you. Do they help you feel better temporarily but leave you feeling worse later? Are they causing harm to yourself or others?

2. Understanding Triggers:

- **Recognize Triggers:** Understand what situations or emotions trigger your need to cope. Identifying triggers can help you anticipate when you might need alternative coping strategies.

- **Explore Underlying Emotions:** Consider the emotions you're experiencing when triggered. Are you feeling stressed, anxious, lonely, or overwhelmed? Understanding the root cause of your emotions can guide you toward healthier coping methods.

3. Explore Alternative Coping Strategies:

- **Healthy Outlets:** Look for healthy activities that can help you cope with stress and difficult emotions. This could include exercise, hobbies, spending time with loved ones, practicing mindfulness or meditation, journaling, or engaging in creative activities.
- **Mindfulness and Relaxation Techniques:** Learn techniques such as deep breathing exercises, progressive muscle relaxation, or visualization to help calm your mind and body during times of stress.
- **Seek assistance**: For assistance and direction, get in touch with friends, family, or mental health specialists. Seeking guidance from others and discussing your emotions with them might offer insightful viewpoints and helpful coping mechanisms.
- **Develop Problem-Solving Skills**: Focus on acquiring efficient problem-solving techniques rather than ignoring or avoiding issues. Divide problems into doable steps and come up with some possible answers.

- **Set Boundaries:** Learn to say no to activities or commitments that add unnecessary stress to your life. Setting boundaries can help you prioritize self-care and reduce overwhelm.
- **Practice Self-compassion:** Develop self-compassion: Be kind and understanding to oneself, especially when things are tough. Recognise your accomplishments and efforts even when things don't go as to plan.

4. Try New Things and Adjust:

• Experiment with Different Techniques: Be willing to try out a variety of coping mechanisms to determine which ones suit you the best. It's crucial to try different things and see what speaks to you since what works for one person might not work for another.

- **Be Patient and Persistent:** Building new coping mechanisms takes time and practice. Be patient with yourself and recognize that change may not happen overnight. Keep trying and adapting until you find strategies that feel effective and sustainable.

5. Reflect and Adjust:

- **Reflect on Your Progress:** Regularly reflect on how your new coping mechanisms

are working for you. Notice any changes in your mood, behavior, and overall well-being.
- **Adjust as Needed:** Be willing to adjust and refine your coping strategies based on what you learn about yourself and your needs over time. It's okay to revisit and modify your approach as you continue to grow and evolve.

Finding alternative coping mechanisms is a journey of self-discovery and self-care. By cultivating self-awareness, exploring healthy outlets, seeking support, and being open to experimentation and growth, you can develop effective strategies for managing stress and navigating life's challenges in a healthier and more resilient way. Remember that it's okay to ask for help along the way and to be gentle with yourself as you learn and grow.

- **Cognitive Behavioral Techniques**

Cognitive Behavioral Therapy (CBT) is a widely practiced and evidence-based approach to psychotherapy that focuses on the connections between thoughts, feelings, and behaviors. Cognitive Behavioral Techniques (CBT techniques) are the specific tools and strategies used within CBT to help individuals identify and modify unhelpful thought patterns, manage emotions, and change behaviors that contribute to psychological distress. Let's look at some key cognitive behavioral techniques:

1. Identifying Automatic Thoughts:

- **Definition:** Automatic thoughts are rapid, spontaneous, and often subconscious thoughts that occur in response to situations or triggers.
- **Technique:** Through self-monitoring and reflection, individuals learn to identify and document their automatic thoughts in various situations.
- **Example:** If someone receives criticism at work, their automatic thought might be, "I'm not good enough," or "I'll never succeed."

2. Challenging Cognitive Distortions:

- **Definition:** Cognitive distortions are irrational and biased ways of thinking that contribute to negative emotions.
- **Technique:** Individuals learn to recognize common cognitive distortions such as black-and-white thinking, catastrophizing, overgeneralization, and personalization.
- **Example:** When faced with rejection, a person might automatically think, "I'm a

failure and always will be," which reflects catastrophizing.

3. Cognitive Restructuring:

- **Definition:** Cognitive restructuring involves challenging and replacing irrational or negative thoughts with more balanced and realistic ones.
- **Technique:** Individuals learn to question the accuracy and validity of their automatic thoughts and replace them with more adaptive interpretations.
- **Example:** Instead of thinking, "I'll never find love because I'm unlovable," they might reframe it as, "I've faced rejection before, but it doesn't mean I'm unworthy of love."

4. Behavioral Experiments:

- **Definition:** Behavioral experiments involve testing the accuracy of beliefs and assumptions through real-life experiences.
- **Technique:** Individuals design experiments to gather evidence for or against their beliefs, allowing them to challenge and modify unhelpful beliefs.
- **Example:** Someone who believes they are socially incompetent might conduct an experiment where they initiate conversations

with strangers to gather evidence about their social skills.

5. Graded Exposure:

- **Definition:** Graded exposure is a technique used to reduce anxiety and fear responses by gradually exposing individuals to feared objects or situations.
- **Technique:** Individuals create a hierarchy of anxiety-provoking situations and systematically confront them, starting with the least distressing and progressing to more challenging scenarios.
- **Example:** A person with a fear of heights might gradually expose themselves to heights by first standing on a small step stool and gradually working up to taller heights.

6. Activity Scheduling:

- **Definition:** Activity scheduling involves structuring daily routines to increase engagement in pleasurable and meaningful activities.
- **Technique:** Individuals identify enjoyable activities and schedule them into their daily lives, even when they don't feel motivated.
- **Example:** Engaging in hobbies, spending time with loved ones, or pursuing personal

interests can be scheduled activities to boost mood and motivation.

7. Relaxation Techniques:

- **Definition:** Relaxation techniques help reduce physiological arousal and promote a sense of calmness and relaxation.
- **Technique:** Individuals practice methods such as deep breathing, progressive muscle relaxation, guided imagery, or mindfulness meditation.
- **Example:** Taking slow, deep breaths during moments of stress or spending a few minutes practicing mindfulness can help induce relaxation and reduce anxiety.

Cognitive behavioral techniques offer practical and effective tools for addressing a wide range of mental health concerns, including depression, anxiety, stress, and interpersonal difficulties. By learning to identify automatic thoughts, challenge cognitive distortions, restructure unhelpful beliefs, conduct behavioral experiments, engage in graded exposure, schedule rewarding activities, and practice relaxation techniques, individuals can develop greater self-awareness, resilience, and emotional well-being. Working with a qualified therapist or mental health professional can provide guidance and support in applying these techniques effectively to address binge eating, specific challenges and achieve therapeutic goals.

Chapter 8

Maintaining Progress and Preventing Relapse

• Staying Committed to Recovery

Staying committed to recovery is a crucial aspect of overcoming challenges related to mental health, substance abuse, eating disorders, trauma, or any other form of psychological distress. Recovery is a journey that requires dedication, resilience, and ongoing effort.

1. Understanding Recovery:

- **Definition:** Recovery is a holistic process of healing and growth that encompasses physical, emotional, mental, and spiritual well-being.
- **Awareness:** Understand that recovery is not just about symptom management but also about improving overall quality of life and functioning.

2. Setting Realistic Goals:

- **Clarity:** Define clear and achievable goals that align with your values and aspirations.
- **Specificity:** Break down long-term goals into smaller, manageable steps to maintain motivation and track progress.

- **Flexibility:** Be open to adjusting goals based on changing circumstances or new insights gained during the recovery journey.

3. Building a Support Network:

- **Connection:** Surround yourself with supportive friends, family members, peers, or professionals who understand and validate your experiences.
- **Community:** Participate in support groups, therapy sessions, or online forums where you can connect with others who are on similar paths of recovery.
- **Accountability:** Share your goals and progress with trusted individuals who can offer encouragement, accountability, and constructive feedback.

4. Practicing Self-Care:

- **Physical Health:** Prioritize activities that promote physical well-being, such as regular exercise, nutritious eating, adequate sleep, and medical check-ups.
- **Emotional Health:** Engage in activities that nurture emotional resilience and self-compassion, such as mindfulness meditation, journaling, creative expression, or therapy.

- **Boundaries:** Establish healthy boundaries to protect your energy and prioritize self-care without feeling guilty or obligated to please others.

5. Developing Coping Skills:

- **Awareness:** Identify triggers, stressors, and negative patterns of thinking or behavior that may undermine your recovery efforts.
- **Skills:** Learn and practice effective coping strategies such as deep breathing, relaxation techniques, cognitive restructuring, problem-solving, and assertive communication.
- **Flexibility:** Experiment with different coping techniques to find what works best for you in various situations and contexts.

6. Embracing Relapse as Part of the Process:

- **Perspective:** Understand that setbacks and relapses are common and natural parts of the recovery journey.
- **Learning Opportunity:** View relapses as opportunities for self-reflection, learning, and growth rather than as signs of failure or weakness.
- **Resilience:** Use relapse as a chance to reassess your strategies, seek additional

support, and recommit to your recovery goals with renewed determination.

7. Celebrating Progress and Milestones:

- **Recognition:** Acknowledge and celebrate your achievements, no matter how small or incremental they may seem.
- **Gratitude:** Cultivate a sense of gratitude for the progress you've made and the lessons you've learned along the way.
- **Self-Compassion:** Practice self-compassion and kindness towards yourself, recognizing that recovery is a process that unfolds over time.

8. Seeking Professional Help When Needed:

- **Awareness:** Recognize when additional support or intervention is necessary to address challenges or barriers to recovery.
- **Accessing Resources:** Reach out to mental health professionals, counselors, therapists, or support services that can provide specialized care and guidance tailored to your needs.
- **Advocacy:** Be an advocate for your own health and well-being by actively seeking out resources and advocating for the support you deserve.

Staying committed to recovery from binge eating involves a combination of self-awareness, support, resilience, and self-care practices. By implementing these strategies and fostering a positive mindset, individuals can navigate the challenges of recovery and cultivate a healthier, more fulfilling life free from the grip of binge eating disorder.

Identifying Warning Signs

Identifying warning signs and implementing strategies to stop binge eating is crucial for individuals who struggle with this behavior. Recurrent episodes of eating a lot of food in a short amount of time while feeling out of control when doing so are the hallmark of binge eating disorder (BED). This is a thorough instruction on spotting warning signs and preventing binge eating or low energy might aid in identifying circumstances when binge eating may occur.

Identifying Warning Signs:

1. **Emotional Triggers:**
   - Binge eating episodes can be brought on by stress, worry, melancholy, loneliness, boredom, or other unpleasant emotions.
   - Identify trends in which episodes of

binge eating are preceded by emotional distress.

2. **Physical Triggers:**
 Restrictive diets, prolonged fasting, or meal skipping can increase appetite and cause binge eating.
• Recognizing physical indicators that indicate acute hunger or low energy might aid in identifying circumstances when binge eating may occur.

3. **Environmental Triggers:**
Parties, social events, and being around a lot of food are examples of settings or circumstances that might lead to binge eating.
• Identify the settings or circumstances that lead to your binge eating episodes and take action to prevent or control them.

4. **Thought Patterns:**
Binge eating behavior can be influenced by negative ideas and attitudes regarding food, body image, and self-worth.
• Be alert for skewed ideas such as self-critical remarks about one's body image or black-and-white reasoning ("I've already eaten one cookie, so I might as well eat the whole box").

5. **Behavioral Patterns:**

Among the behavioral signs of binge eating are eating in secret, hiding food wrappers, or experiencing guilt or embarrassment afterward.
• Keep an eye on eating patterns and behaviors to spot trends linked to episodes of binge eating.

Strategies to Stop Binge Eating:

1. **Develop Awareness:**
    - Keep a food diary to track eating patterns, emotions, and triggers associated with binge eating episodes.
    - Practice mindfulness techniques to increase awareness of physical sensations, emotions, and thought patterns related to eating.
2. **Identify Triggers:**
    - Recognize and understand the triggers that lead to binge eating episodes, including emotional, physical, and environmental factors.
    - Work with a therapist or counselor to explore underlying emotions and experiences contributing to binge eating behavior.
3. **Develop Coping Strategies:**
    - Learn healthy coping mechanisms to manage stress, anxiety, and negative emotions without resorting to food.

- Engage in activities such as exercise, meditation, deep breathing, journaling, or spending time with supportive friends and family members.

4. **Practice Mindful Eating:**
   - Focus on the sensory experience of eating, including taste, texture, and aroma, to enhance awareness and enjoyment of food.
   - Slow down during meals, chew food thoroughly, and savor each bite to prevent mindless overeating.

5. **Challenge Distorted Thoughts:**
   - Challenge negative thoughts and beliefs about food, body image, and self-worth with rational, positive affirmations.
   - Replace negative self-talk with compassionate and realistic statements that promote self-acceptance and self-care.

6. **Seek Professional Help:**
   - Consider seeking support from a therapist, counselor, or registered dietitian who specializes in treating binge eating disorder.
   - Cognitive-behavioral therapy (CBT), dialectical behavior therapy (DBT), and mindfulness-based interventions

are evidence-based approaches for managing binge eating behavior.

7. **Establish Healthy Eating Habits:**
   - Eat regular, balanced meals and snacks throughout the day to maintain stable blood sugar levels and prevent extreme hunger.
   - Include a variety of nutrient-dense foods such as fruits, vegetables, lean proteins, whole grains, and healthy fats in your diet.

8. **Build a Support Network:**
   - Surround yourself with supportive individuals who understand your struggles and provide encouragement, empathy, and accountability.
   - Join a support group or online community for individuals recovering from binge eating disorder to share experiences, insights, and resources.

Stopping binge eating requires patience, self-awareness, and a commitment to adopting healthy coping strategies and behaviors. By identifying warning signs, developing effective coping mechanisms, and seeking support when needed, individuals can take proactive steps towards overcoming binge eating disorder and improving their overall well-being.

- ## **Strategies for Long-Term Success**

A mix of behavioral, lifestyle, and psychological techniques are used in long-term binge eating prevention strategies to address the root causes of the illness and encourage long-lasting modifications to eating patterns and coping techniques. This is a comprehensive guide on long-term successful tactics for overcoming binge eating:

1. Recognize Patterns and Triggers:

Self-knowledge: Record your binge eating events in a notebook, noting any feelings, circumstances, or thoughts that may have preceded the binge.

Determine patterns: Acknowledge recurrent triggers and behaviors linked to binge eating, such as psychological discomfort, severe dieting, or particular food desires.

2. Develop Coping Skills:

- **Healthy coping mechanisms:** Learn alternative ways to manage stress, anxiety, and negative emotions without resorting to binge eating. This could include mindfulness, deep breathing exercises, journaling, or engaging in enjoyable activities.

- **Emotional regulation:** Practice recognizing and accepting emotions without judgment, and develop strategies for processing and expressing feelings in constructive ways.

3. Practice Mindful Eating:

- **Sensory awareness:** Pay attention to the taste, texture, and smell of food while eating, and savor each bite mindfully.
- **Eating environment:** Create a peaceful and distraction-free eating environment, focusing on the meal rather than television, computer, or phone screens.

4. Establish Regular Eating Patterns:

- **Structured meals:** Eat balanced meals at regular intervals throughout the day to prevent extreme hunger and stabilize blood sugar levels.
- **Include all food groups:** Ensure meals contain a variety of nutrient-dense foods, including fruits, vegetables, lean proteins, whole grains, and healthy fats.

5. Challenge Negative Thoughts:

- **Cognitive restructuring:** Challenge and reframe negative thoughts and beliefs about food, body image, and self-worth. Replace self-critical thoughts with compassionate and realistic affirmations.

- **Positive self-talk:** Cultivate a mindset of self-compassion and acceptance, acknowledging progress and setbacks without judgment.

6. Seek Professional Support:

- **Therapy:** Consider working with a therapist or counselor who specializes in eating disorders, such as cognitive-behavioral therapy (CBT), dialectical behavior therapy (DBT), or interpersonal therapy (IPT).
- **Nutritional counseling:** To create a sustainable and well-balanced eating plan that suits your needs and tastes, speak with a qualified dietician.
Medication: To treat underlying emotional disorders or co-occurring problems that contribute to binge eating, doctors may occasionally prescribe medication.

7. Build a Support Network:

- **Peer support:** Connect with others who have experienced or are recovering from binge eating disorder through support groups, online forums, or community organizations.

- **Family and friends:** Educate loved ones about binge eating disorder and enlist their support in your recovery journey. Communicate openly about your needs and challenges.

8. Practice Self-Care:

- **Prioritize sleep:** Aim for consistent and restful sleep each night to support overall health and well-being.
- **Regular physical activity:** Engage in enjoyable forms of exercise that promote physical and mental wellness, such as walking, yoga, or dancing.
- **Stress management:** Incorporate relaxation techniques and self-care practices into your daily routine to reduce stress and enhance resilience.

9. Set Realistic Goals:

- **Gradual progress:** Set achievable goals for behavior change and celebrate small victories along the way. Be patient and compassionate with yourself during periods of challenge or setback.
- **Focus on sustainability:** Emphasize long-term habits and lifestyle changes rather than short-term fixes or restrictive diets.

10. Stay Committed to Recovery:

- **Persistence:** Recognize that recovery from binge eating disorder is a journey that may involve ups and downs. Stay committed to your goals and remain resilient in the face of setbacks.
- **Professional monitoring:** Regularly check in with your treatment team to assess progress, address any emerging concerns, and make adjustments to your treatment plan as needed.

By integrating these strategies into your daily life and seeking support from qualified professionals and supportive networks, you can cultivate lasting changes and achieve long-term success in overcoming binge eating disorder. Remember that recovery is possible, and you deserve to live a life free from the burden of disordered eating.

Thank you!

Thank you for your purchase. If you enjoyed this book, please kindly consider dropping us a review.